Preface

Introduction to the Book

This book is crafted to provide a comprehensive understanding of the nursing profession, a field often misunderstood and underestimated in its diversity and depth. Many individuals are drawn to nursing, intrigued by its promise of care and service, yet they lack a clear picture of what the nursing world truly encompasses. This book aims to demystify the profession, offering insights into the myriad roles and opportunities that nursing presents. Whether your interest lies in the high-intensity environment of the ICU or the strategic realm of nursing management, this guide serves as a beacon, illuminating the path to aligning your passion with a suitable nursing career.

The Evolving Role of Nursing in Healthcare

Nursing has undergone a remarkable evolution, expanding far beyond the walls of traditional medical centers. Today's nurses find themselves in a variety of settings – from the esteemed corridors of the White House to the dynamic arenas of the military, and even in the skies as flight nurses. This evolution is a testament to the adaptability and critical importance of nurses in healthcare. The book explores how nursing serves as a foundation for diverse career paths, enabling practitioners to reach new heights and broaden their impact in healthcare.

Purpose and Audience of the Book

The primary goal of this book is to provide an in-depth understanding of the nursing profession, catering to a wide audience. It is an invaluable resource for current nursing students seeking direction, for those contemplating a career in nursing, and equally for those who are at a crossroads, considering various specializations within the field. Through this book, readers will gain a clearer perspective of nursing's vast landscape, helping them make informed decisions about their professional journeys in healthcare.

Chapter 1: Navigating Hospital Nursing Units

Hospitals are complex institutions with various specialized units, each catering to different types of medical needs. Here's a breakdown of the common units you'll find in a hospital:

Emergency Room (ER) or Emergency Department (ED)

The first point of contact for patients with urgent medical conditions.

Equipped to handle a wide range of emergencies, from trauma to cardiac events.

Staffed by physicians, nurses, and support staff trained in emergency medicine.

Patients may be transferred from ED to various units depending on their condition – ICU for critical cases, Med-Surg for less critical issues, or specialized units like Cardiology or Neurology if needed.

The Emergency Room (ER)

The ER, known for its fast-paced and unpredictable nature, is the frontline of medical urgency. Here, nurses encounter a wide spectrum of conditions, from minor injuries to life-threatening emergencies.

Role of ER Nurses: ER nurses are trained to quickly assess patient needs, stabilize conditions, and administer immediate care. Their responsibilities include triaging patients based on the severity of their conditions, providing emergency treatments, and coordinating with doctors for further medical interventions. These nurses must be adept at handling everything from trauma to cardiac arrests, often making split-second decisions that can save lives.

Skills and Environment: The ER environment demands nurses who are not only clinically skilled but also capable of managing stress and rapid change. They must possess excellent critical thinking skills, emotional stability, and the ability to work effectively in a team. The ER is a hub of constant activity, requiring nurses to be adaptable and resilient.

Patient Care Pathways in the ER

In the ER, patient care pathways are critical for ensuring that each patient receives timely and appropriate treatment. The pathway typically starts with triage, where nurses assess the urgency of a patient's condition. Following this, patients are either treated and discharged, admitted to the hospital, or referred to specialized units for further care.

Triage: Upon arrival, ER nurses assess patients' conditions, determining who needs immediate care. This rapid evaluation is crucial in a setting where minutes can make a difference.

Treatment and Stabilization: ER nurses provide initial treatment, which could range from wound care to life-saving resuscitation efforts. Their role is to stabilize patients for further care, be it in the ER or elsewhere in the hospital.

Admission or Referral: Patients whose conditions require extended hospital care are admitted to relevant units, such as the ICU for critically ill patients or the Medical-Surgical unit for those needing ongoing treatment. Some patients may be referred to specialized units like Cardiology or Neurology based on their specific needs.

Discharge or Transfer: Patients who do not require hospitalization are discharged with instructions for follow-up care. In some cases, patients might be transferred to other facilities for specialized treatment or rehabilitation.

Intensive Care Unit (ICU):

Provides intensive treatment and monitoring for critically ill patients.

ICU nurses are trained in advanced life support and critical care.

Equipped with advanced medical technology.

Staff includes critical care nurses, intensivists (physicians specialized in critical care), and various specialists depending on the patient's condition.

Patients often transfer from ICU to Step-Down or Med-Surg units as they stabilize.

Intensive Care Unit (ICU)

The ICU represents the pinnacle of critical care in the hospital, catering to patients with life-threatening illnesses or injuries.

Role of ICU Nurses: Nurses in the ICU are specialized in managing complex and severe health conditions. They provide continuous care and monitoring for patients on life support systems, such as ventilators and intravenous infusions. These nurses are experts in assessing critical changes in patient conditions and implementing quick interventions.

Skills and Environment: The ICU demands nurses who are skilled in advanced medical technology and possess a deep understanding of complex pathophysiology. The environment is highly demanding, requiring nurses to be detail-oriented, emotionally strong, and capable of making crucial decisions under pressure.

Step-Down or Progressive Care Unit

For patients who no longer need ICU care but still require more attention than provided on a general Med-Surg floor.

Nurses here are skilled in monitoring patients in transition.

Patients often transfer to Med-Surg or specialized units as they continue to recover.

Post-Anesthesia Care Unit (PACU)

Provides care for patients recovering from anesthesia post-surgery.

PACU nurses monitor patients' vital signs, pain levels, and readiness to leave PACU.

Patients are transferred here from the OR and then to ICU, Med-Surg, or specialized units based on their post-operative condition.

Operating Room (OR)

A sterile environment where surgical procedures are performed.

Includes surgeons, anesthesiologists, surgical nurses, and technicians.

Patients come from various units (ICU, Med-Surg, specialized units like Cardiology) for surgeries and are typically transferred to Post-Anesthesia Care Unit (PACU) or directly to ICU or Med-Surg units post-surgery.

Maternity Ward or Obstetrics (OB) Unit

Specializes in care for pregnant women and childbirth.

Includes labor and delivery rooms, postpartum units for mother and newborn care.

Staff includes obstetricians, midwives, neonatal nurses.

New mothers and babies may transfer to a general room in the OB unit after delivery or go home.

Neonatal Intensive Care Unit (NICU)

Provides care for premature or critically ill newborns.

Equipped with incubators and specialized equipment.

Staffed by neonatologists, neonatal nurses, and respiratory therapists.

Pediatric Unit

Specialized care for infants, children, and adolescents.

Pediatricians and pediatric nurses provide care tailored to younger patients.

Infants may transfer from the NICU, while older children might come from the ED or Med-Surg units.

Medical-Surgical Unit (Med-Surg):

The largest unit in most hospitals.

Provides care for patients recovering from surgery or with various medical conditions.

Staffed by general surgeons, physicians, and medical nurses.

Patients may transfer to specialized units (like Cardiology) if specific conditions arise, or to Rehabilitation for recovery and therapy.

Cardiology Unit

Specializes in heart-related conditions.

Includes cardiac monitoring equipment.

Staffed by cardiologists, cardiac nurses, and technicians.

Patients may transfer to specialized units (like Cardiology) if specific conditions arise, or to Rehabilitation for recovery and therapy.

Oncology Unit

Dedicated to cancer patients.

Offers chemotherapy, radiation therapy, and other treatments.

Staffed by oncologists, oncology nurses, and support staff.

Patients may come from Med-Surg units or directly from outpatient settings.

Radiology Department

Provides imaging services like X-rays, MRIs, CT scans.

Radiologists and radiology technicians operate the equipment and interpret results.

Laboratory

Conducts medical tests to diagnose and monitor diseases.

Staffed by pathologists, medical technologists, and lab technicians.

Rehabilitation Unit:

Offers therapy (physical, occupational, speech) for patients recovering from injuries or surgeries.

Staffed by therapists, rehab nurses, and physiatrists.

Psychiatric Unit

Provides care for patients with mental health disorders.

Includes psychiatrists, psychologists, psychiatric nurses, and therapists.

Palliative Care Unit

Focuses on providing relief from the symptoms and stress of serious illness.

Aims to improve quality of life for both the patient and the family.

Geriatric Unit

Specializes in the care of elderly patients.

Addresses complex health issues related to aging.

Patients may come from Med-Surg, Rehabilitation, or directly from the ED.

Outpatient Surgery Nursing Unit

Cares for patients undergoing surgeries that don't require overnight hospitalization.

Nurses assist in pre-operative preparation and post-operative recovery.

Patients usually return home the same day after recovery under the nurse's care.

Cardiac Catheterization Lab Nursing Unit

Assists with procedures like cardiac catheterizations and angioplasties.

Nurses prepare patients, assist during procedures, and provide post-procedure care.

Patients often come from the ED, Cardiology, or ICU and may return to those units or be admitted to Med-Surg for further care.

Endoscopy Nursing Unit

Supports procedures involving the gastrointestinal tract, like upper endoscopies or bronchoscopies.

Nurses assist with patient preparation, procedure support, and post-procedure monitoring.

Patients typically come from GI, Med-Surg, or outpatient and return or are admitted based on the outcome.

Pre-Operative Nursing Unit

Prepares patients for surgery.

Nurses conduct pre-operative assessments and patient education.

Patients are transferred here from various hospital units or outpatient settings before moving to the OR.

Ambulatory Care Nursing Unit

Provides care for patients receiving treatments or undergoing minor procedures that don't require hospitalization.

Nurses manage a wide range of care, from IV therapy to wound care.

Patients come from outpatient settings and return home the same day.

Infusion Therapy Nursing Unit

Specializes in administering medications and fluids intravenously, such as chemotherapy.

Nurses monitor patients during infusions and manage any reactions.

Patients may come from Oncology, Med-Surg, or outpatient settings.

Each of these units plays a critical role in patient care, and nurses are essential in ensuring smooth transitions and continuity of care throughout a patient's hospital journey. Coordination among units, clear communication, and comprehensive care planning are vital for effective patient care in these diverse settings.

Chapter 2

Diverse Career Paths for Nurses Beyond the Hospital

Nurses have a wide range of employment opportunities outside of traditional hospital settings. These roles often allow nurses to work in diverse environments, providing care in different contexts or focusing on specific populations. Here are some places outside the hospital where nurses can work:

Primary Care Clinics

Provide general health care services.

Nurses perform routine checks, administer vaccinations, and assist with minor procedures.

Nurses in primary care clinics and specialist doctor's offices provide comprehensive healthcare services, ranging from routine health checks to assisting with specialized medical procedures. They play a vital role in patient education, chronic disease management, and preventive healthcare.

Specialist Doctor's Offices

Offices of healthcare specialists like dermatologists, cardiologists, or pediatricians.

Nurses assist with specific medical procedures and patient care relevant to the specialty.

Home Health Care

Provide medical care in patients' homes.

Nurses manage medication, wound care, and monitor health status for chronically ill, elderly, or post-operative patients.

Home health care nurses provide medical care in patients' homes, catering to those who are chronically ill, elderly, or recovering from surgery. They manage medications, wound care, and monitor the overall health status of patients, playing a crucial role in allowing patients to recover in the comfort of their homes.

Nursing Homes/Long-Term Care Facilities

Care for elderly or disabled individuals.

Nurses monitor health, administer medications, and manage chronic conditions.

Nursing in long-term care facilities and nursing homes involves caring for elderly or disabled individuals. Nurses in these settings manage medications, assist with daily living activities, and monitor residents' health, focusing on enhancing their quality of life.

Schools and Universities

Provide health services in educational institutions.

School nurses handle emergencies, manage chronic illnesses in students, and promote health education.

Community Health Centers

Offer health services in community settings, often focusing on underserved populations.

Nurses provide care, education, and outreach on various health issues.

Occupational Health in Business and Industry

Work in corporate or industrial settings.

Nurses manage workplace injuries, conduct health screenings, and promote workplace wellness programs.

Occupational health nurses are employed in business and industrial settings. They focus on employee health and safety, manage workplace injuries, conduct health screenings, and develop wellness programs.

Public Health Departments

Focus on community-wide health initiatives.

Nurses participate in public health campaigns, disease prevention, and health education.

Public health nurses work in community health centers and government agencies, focusing on public health initiatives. They are involved in disease prevention, health promotion, community education, and managing public health crises.

Military and Government Agencies

Serve in branches of the military or government entities like the Veterans Administration.

Nurses provide care to service members, veterans, and government employees.

Military nurses serve in various branches of the armed forces, providing healthcare to military personnel and their families. They may work in military hospitals, clinics, or field units and have the opportunity to serve in various locations around the world.

Research and Pharmaceutical Companies

Involved in clinical research and trials.

Nurses monitor patient responses to treatments and collect data for research studies.

Nurses in research contribute to medical and healthcare knowledge, often working in research institutions or academia. Nurse educators, on the other hand, are crucial in training the next generation of nurses, working in universities, colleges, and training programs.

Telehealth Services

Provide nursing care remotely via phone or internet.

Nurses offer consultation, health advice, and triage services.

Telehealth nurses provide care remotely via digital platforms. They offer consultation, health advice, and triage services, playing a critical role in increasing healthcare accessibility.

Telehealth nurses provide care remotely via digital platforms. They offer consultation, health advice, and triage services, playing a critical role in increasing healthcare accessibility.

Hospice Care

Provide end-of-life care.

Nurses manage pain relief, provide emotional support, and assist families during the palliative care process.

School Nursing

School nurses work in educational settings, providing health services to students. They manage emergencies, oversee medication administration, and play a key role in health education and promoting a healthy school environment.

Travel Nursing

Temporary assignments in various locations, often in response to specific healthcare shortages.

Nurses have the opportunity to work in multiple settings, both urban and rural.

Freelance or Consultancy Work

Independent nursing consultants provide expert advice on healthcare systems, policies, or nursing practices.

Health Insurance Companies

Work in case management or as claims advisers.

Nurses review medical claims, provide health advice to policyholders, and help manage care plans.

Non-Governmental Organizations (NGOs)

Work in humanitarian and global health settings.

Nurses provide care in crisis zones, participate in health campaigns, and work on global health initiatives.

These roles allow nurses to apply their skills in various contexts, impacting health and wellness in communities, schools, workplaces, and beyond. The diversity in nursing roles outside hospitals reflects the versatility and adaptability of the nursing profession.

High-Adventure Nursing Careers: Flight and Military Nursing

Nursing is a versatile profession that offers a wide range of career paths beyond traditional hospital and clinical settings. Two exciting and dynamic fields for nurses are flight nursing and military nursing:

Flight Nurse

Role and Responsibilities: Flight nurses provide critical care in air medical transport settings, such as helicopters or fixed-wing aircraft. They are responsible for stabilizing and caring for patients during medical evacuations or transfers between facilities. This includes trauma victims, critical care transfers, and patients needing emergency medical attention.

Skills and Training: Flight nurses must have specialized training in critical care, emergency nursing, and must be able to make quick decisions in high-stress, unpredictable environments. They typically need several years of experience in critical care or emergency nursing before transitioning to flight nursing.

Certifications: Many flight nurses hold certifications like Critical Care Registered Nurse (CCRN), Certified Emergency Nurse (CEN), or Flight Registered Nurse (CFRN). Advanced Cardiac Life Support (ACLS) and Pediatric Advanced Life Support (PALS) are also essential.

Work Environment: The work environment is highly variable and can be physically demanding. Flight nurses must be prepared to work in confined spaces and under challenging conditions, including extreme weather, and varying altitudes.

Military Nurse

Role and Responsibilities: Military nurses serve in different branches of the armed forces, including the Army, Navy, and Air Force. They provide healthcare to military personnel, veterans, and their families. This can include working in combat zones, military hospitals, and on bases around the world.

Skills and Training: Military nurses need to be adaptable, resilient, and able to handle high-pressure situations. They must be prepared for deployment and providing care in diverse settings, from field hospitals to state-of-the-art medical facilities.

Certifications and Requirements: While military nurses are primarily registered nurses, additional certifications relevant to trauma and emergency care can be beneficial. They must also meet the physical and mental fitness standards required for military service.

Work Environment: The work environment can range from standard medical facilities to field units in conflict zones. Military nurses may also engage in humanitarian missions, providing care in disaster-stricken or underserved areas globally.

Career Development: Serving as a military nurse can offer unique opportunities for career advancement and specialization. The military also provides avenues for further education and training in various nursing specialties.

Both flight nursing and military nursing are careers that require not only nursing skills but also physical endurance, emotional resilience, and the ability to work under challenging and sometimes extreme conditions. These roles offer unique opportunities to serve in critical and high-impact situations, making a significant difference in the lives of patients in need of urgent medical care.

Chapter 3

The Impactful World of Nursing in Healthcare Administration

Nurses can also find fulfilling careers in administrative roles, where they leverage their clinical expertise to improve healthcare systems, policies, and practices. Here's a look at some administrative roles suitable for nurses:

Nurse Manager or Head Nurse

Oversee nursing staff in healthcare facilities.

Responsibilities include staff management, scheduling, and maintaining quality patient care standards.

Clinical Nurse Leader (CNL)

A relatively new role designed to improve the quality of patient care outcomes.

CNLs oversee the integration of care for a specific set of patients and manage care coordination.

Nurse Administrator

Involved in the managerial and administrative aspects of nursing services.

Responsibilities include budgeting, policy development, and facility management.

Nurse Educator or Clinical Instructor

Work in academic settings to train and educate future nurses.

Responsibilities include curriculum development, teaching, and mentorship.

Chief Nursing Officer (CNO) or Director of Nursing

Top-level executive responsible for overseeing all nursing staff and operations within a healthcare organization.

Focus on strategic planning, policy implementation, and maintaining nursing standards.

Healthcare Consultant

Provide expert advice to healthcare organizations on improving efficiency, compliance, and patient outcomes.

Often work with healthcare facilities to develop and implement new policies or programs.

Nurse Informaticist

Specialize in managing healthcare data and information systems.

Combine nursing knowledge with information technology skills to improve patient care delivery.

Quality Improvement Coordinator

Focus on enhancing the quality and effectiveness of healthcare services.

Responsibilities include data analysis, process improvement initiatives, and compliance monitoring.

Case Manager

Coordinate long-term care for patients, particularly those with chronic illnesses or complex medical needs.

Focus on ensuring patients receive appropriate care while managing healthcare costs.

Nurse Policy Analyst

Work with governmental agencies or healthcare organizations to develop policies affecting healthcare delivery.

Responsibilities include policy research, analysis, and advocacy.

Nurse Lobbyist or Advocate

Work to influence healthcare policies at local, state, or national levels.

Represent healthcare interests, particularly nursing perspectives, in policy discussions.

Research Administrator

Oversee nursing research programs, including budgeting, compliance, and staff management.

Ensure research projects adhere to ethical guidelines and regulatory standards.

Risk Management Officer

Focus on identifying, evaluating, and minimizing risks within healthcare settings.

Develop strategies to improve patient safety and reduce potential liabilities.

These administrative roles allow nurses to impact patient care on a systemic level, utilizing their clinical background to inform decisions and policies. Nurses in administrative positions play a crucial role in shaping the healthcare landscape, driving improvements in patient care, efficiency, and healthcare delivery methods.

Expanded Roles and Responsibilities

Strategic Planning and Implementation

Nurses in administrative roles are pivotal in strategic planning and the implementation of healthcare policies and practices. They bring a practical, hands-on perspective to policy development, ensuring that new protocols not only meet regulatory standards but are also feasible and beneficial from a caregiver's viewpoint. For example, a Chief Nursing Officer (CNO) might spearhead initiatives to integrate cutting-edge technology in patient care, enhancing both efficiency and outcomes.

Enhancing Patient Care through Innovation

Nurse Administrators and Managers play a vital role in innovating patient care practices. Their firsthand experience with patient care enables them to identify areas for improvement and advocate for the adoption of new, evidence-based practices. They might lead projects to redesign patient flow, reduce wait times, and enhance the overall patient experience within a healthcare facility.

Quality and Safety Oversight

Quality Improvement Coordinators and Risk Management Officers are tasked with the critical responsibility of overseeing patient safety and the quality of care. By analyzing incident reports, patient feedback, and clinical data, they identify trends and develop strategies to mitigate risks, enhancing the safety and quality of patient care. Their work ensures that healthcare facilities not only comply with regulatory requirements but also strive for excellence in patient care.

Integrating Technology and Healthcare

Nurse Informaticists represent a bridge between clinical care and information technology, playing a crucial role in the adoption and optimization of electronic health records (EHRs) and other healthcare IT systems. Their understanding of clinical workflows, combined with technical skills, enables them to tailor IT solutions that support efficient and effective patient care. They are instrumental in training staff on new systems, ensuring that technology serves as a tool to enhance, rather than hinder, patient care.

Education and Mentorship

Nurse Educators and Clinical Instructors are at the forefront of preparing the next generation of nurses, shaping the future of healthcare through education. They not only impart critical knowledge and skills but also instill values of compassion, ethics, and professionalism in their students. By mentoring novice nurses and facilitating continuing education for experienced staff, they ensure that the nursing workforce remains competent, resilient, and ready to meet the challenges of modern healthcare.

Policy Advocacy and Community Health

Nurse Policy Analysts, Lobbyists, and Advocates work tirelessly to influence healthcare policies at various levels. By representing the nursing perspective in policy discussions, they ensure that healthcare legislation and regulations address the needs of both patients and healthcare providers. Their advocacy supports initiatives aimed at improving community health, such as access to care, public health campaigns, and social determinants of health.

Research and Evidence-Based Practice

Research Administrators oversee nursing research, promoting evidence-based practices that enhance patient outcomes. They ensure that research projects are conducted ethically and yield actionable insights that can be translated into clinical practice. Their work supports the continuous advancement of nursing science, contributing to the development of more effective, efficient, and patient-centered healthcare services.

Nurses in administrative roles leverage their clinical expertise and leadership abilities to make substantial contributions to healthcare administration. By overseeing staff, developing policies, implementing innovations, and advocating for patient-centered care, they play a crucial role in shaping the healthcare landscape. Their work ensures that healthcare organizations not only meet today's challenges but are also prepared for tomorrow's opportunities, ultimately driving improvements in patient care, efficiency, and healthcare delivery methods. Through their diverse roles and responsibilities, these nurse leaders exemplify the profound impact nursing can have beyond the bedside, influencing systemic changes that benefit patients, healthcare teams, and communities at large.

Chapter 4

Specialized Nursing Certifications and Their Professional Significance

There are numerous nursing certifications available, each tailored to specific areas of nursing practice. Here's a list of some common nursing certifications and the nursing units or specialties where they are most relevant.

Certified Pediatric Nurse (CPN)

Relevant to: Pediatric Nursing Units, Pediatric Clinics, Pediatric Intensive Care Units (PICU).

Focused on caring for infants, children, and adolescents. Pediatric nurses must be adept at communicating with younger patients and understanding their unique needs.

Oncology Certified Nurse (OCN)

Relevant to: Oncology Units, Cancer Treatment Centers, Hospice Care.

Specializes in caring for cancer patients. Oncology nurses administer chemotherapy, manage symptoms, and provide emotional support to patients and families.

Critical Care Registered Nurse (CCRN)

Relevant to: Intensive Care Units (ICU), Critical Care Units, Emergency Departments.

Involves caring for patients with life-threatening conditions, typically in ICU settings. Critical care nurses must be skilled in advanced life support and rapid decision-making.

Family Nurse Practitioner (FNP-BC)

Relevant to: Primary Care Clinics, Family Practice, Outpatient Care Centers.

Certified Emergency Nurse (CEN)

Relevant to: Emergency Departments, Trauma Centers, Urgent Care Clinics.

Neonatal Intensive Care Nursing (RNC-NIC)

Relevant to: Neonatal Intensive Care Units (NICU), Perinatal Centers.

Certified Nurse Midwife (CNM)

Relevant to: Maternity Wards, Obstetrics and Gynecology Units, Birthing Centers.

Certified Nephrology Nurse (CNN)

Relevant to: Dialysis Centers, Nephrology Units, Renal Units.

Certified Registered Nurse Anesthetist (CRNA)

Relevant to: Operating Rooms, Surgical Centers, Pain Management Clinics.

Orthopedic Nurse Certified (ONC)

Relevant to: Orthopedic Units, Rehabilitation Centers, Sports Medicine Clinics.

Certified Medical-Surgical Registered Nurse (CMSRN)

Relevant to: Medical-Surgical Units, General Wards, Inpatient Care Units.

Cardiac Vascular Nursing Certification (RN-BC)

Relevant to: Cardiology Units, Cardiac Catheterization Labs, Heart Failure Clinics.

Certified Psychiatric Mental Health Nurse (PMHN)

Relevant to: Psychiatric Units, Mental Health Centers, Substance Abuse Programs.

Certified Diabetes Educator (CDE)

Relevant to: Endocrinology Units, Diabetes Education Centers, Primary Care Clinics.

Certified Perioperative Nurse (CNOR)

Relevant to: Operating Rooms, Surgical Units, Day Surgery Centers.

Certified Wound Care Nurse (CWCN)

Relevant to: Wound Care Centers, Long-term Care Facilities, Home Health Care.

Gerontological Nursing Certification (RN-BC)

Relevant to: Geriatric Units, Long-term Care Facilities, Senior Health Clinics.

Certified Hospice and Palliative Nurse (CHPN)

Relevant to: Hospice Care, Palliative Care Units, Home Health Services.

Certified Infection Control Nurse (CIC)

Relevant to: Infection Control Departments, Public Health Units, Epidemiology Departments.

Nurse Informatics Certification (RN-BC)

Relevant to: Healthcare Informatics, Health Information Technology Departments, Research Institutions.

Certified Neuroscience Registered Nurse (CNRN)

Relevant to: Neurological Units, Neurosurgical Units, Stroke Centers, Intensive Care Units (especially those with a focus on neurological care), and Rehabilitation Units specializing in neurological recovery.

This certification is offered by the American Board of Neuroscience Nursing (ABNN).

CNRN certification demonstrates specialized knowledge in caring for patients with neurological trauma and disorders, such as strokes, brain injuries, spinal cord injuries, and neurological diseases like Parkinson's, Alzheimer's, and epilepsy.

Nurses seeking CNRN certification typically need to have experience in a neuro-focused clinical setting and must pass a certification examination that covers a wide range of neurological conditions and care practices.

Additionally, for nurses working in stroke care, there is the Stroke *Certified Registered Nurse (SCRN)* certification, also offered by the ABNN. This certification is specifically focused on stroke care and is relevant to units such as stroke centers, emergency departments, and ICUs where stroke patients are frequently treated.

Both the CNRN and SCRN certifications are highly valuable for nurses who wish to demonstrate their expertise in neurology and neurosurgery nursing and are instrumental in advancing their careers in these specialized fields.

Each certification requires specific qualifications, such as clinical experience in the specialty area, and passing a certification exam. These certifications not only validate a nurse's expertise in a particular area but also often lead to career advancement, specialization, and increased responsibility within their respective fields.

Exploring a Unique Field: Nursing Informatics

Nursing Informatics is a specialty that merges nursing science with information management and analytical sciences. It plays a crucial role in enhancing patient care through the optimization of information processes.

Role and Scope of Nursing Informatics

Nursing informaticists focus on improving the management of information and communications in nursing to increase efficiency, reduce costs, and enhance the quality of patient care.

They work in various settings, including hospitals, healthcare organizations, research institutions, and technology companies.

Skills and Knowledge Base

Professionals in this field require a combination of nursing knowledge and proficiency in information technology.

 Key skills include data management, health information technology (HIT) systems analysis, and project management, alongside a strong foundation in clinical nursing practice.

Certification Process

To specialize in informatics, nurses typically pursue additional education, such as a graduate degree in nursing informatics or a related field.

Certification, like the Informatics Nursing Certification (RN-BC) offered by the American Nurses Credentialing Center (ANCC), involves a combination of educational requirements, clinical informatics experience, and passing an examination.

Importance of Informatics Certification

Certification in nursing informatics validates a nurse's expertise in this unique intersection of healthcare and technology.

It equips nurses to play a pivotal role in developing and implementing HIT systems that improve patient outcomes and streamline healthcare delivery.

Informatics nurses are crucial in the evolution of healthcare technology, ensuring that technological advancements align with clinical needs and enhance patient care quality.

The Path to Specialization

The journey to nursing specialization typically involves gaining experience in the desired area, pursuing advanced education if needed, and obtaining the relevant certification. It's a path marked by continual learning and professional growth.

Chapter 5

Advanced Practice Nursing: Expanding Roles and Responsibilities

Introduction

This chapter delves into the realm of Advanced Practice Nursing (APN), a sector characterized by greater autonomy, specialized skills, and advanced educational qualifications. The chapter explores the various roles within APN, including Nurse Practitioners, Clinical Nurse Specialists, Nurse Anesthetists, and Nurse Midwives, highlighting their expanded scope of practice and the vital roles they play in the healthcare system.

Nurse Practitioners (NPs)

Overview: NPs are registered nurses with advanced academic and clinical experience.

Roles and Responsibilities: They provide a range of healthcare services, including diagnosis, treatment, and management of acute and chronic conditions. NPs often serve as primary care providers.

Specializations: The section discusses various NP specialties, such as Family, Pediatric, Geriatric, and Psychiatric-Mental Health Nurse Practitioners.

Impact on Healthcare: The role of NPs in improving access to healthcare, particularly in underserved areas, is emphasized.

Clinical Nurse Specialists (CNSs)

Overview: CNSs are experts in a specific area of nursing practice, such as a population, setting, disease, type of care, or type of problem.

Roles and Responsibilities: They provide direct patient care, influence care outcomes by providing expert consultation for nursing staffs and lead organizational change.

Specializations: Examples include CNSs in Oncology, Cardiology, and Psychiatric-Mental Health.

Contribution to Nursing Practice: The section highlights how CNSs enhance the quality of nursing practice through clinical expertise, research, and education.

Nurse Anesthetists (CRNAs)

Overview: Certified Registered Nurse Anesthetists (CRNAs) specialize in the administration of anesthesia.

Roles and Responsibilities: CRNAs manage anesthesia care for patients undergoing surgical, diagnostic, therapeutic, and obstetrical procedures. They are responsible for pre-anesthetic assessment, anesthesia induction, maintenance, and emergence.

Work Settings: The diverse settings in which CRNAs practice, including hospitals, outpatient surgical centers, and rural clinics, are discussed.

Nurse Midwives (CNMs)

Overview: Certified Nurse-Midwives provide comprehensive women's health care, particularly around maternity.

Roles and Responsibilities: CNMs offer prenatal care, labor and delivery support, postpartum care, and gynecological services. They focus on holistic, patient-centered care.

Scope of Practice: The section explores the broad scope of CNMs, emphasizing their role in promoting natural childbirth and providing family-centered maternity care.

Deep Dive into Advanced Practice Roles

Nurse Practitioners (NPs): Pioneers in Primary Care

NPs stand at the forefront of primary care, offering holistic and patient-centered services. Beyond their clinical roles, NPs are increasingly involved in healthcare reform, advocating for patient rights and access to care. Their unique position allows them to address healthcare disparities, especially in rural and underserved communities where they may be the primary, and sometimes only, healthcare providers. The evolution of NP roles, including their authority to prescribe medications and their ability to perform procedures independently in some states, reflects the growing trust in their expertise and the necessity of their expanded scope in addressing the healthcare needs of diverse populations.

Clinical Nurse Specialists (CNSs): Experts in Specialized Care

CNSs, with their deep expertise in specific areas of healthcare, are instrumental in elevating clinical practices through evidence-based interventions. Their work, often behind the scenes, includes developing nursing protocols that enhance patient safety, improve clinical outcomes, and reduce costs. The challenges they face include navigating the complexities of healthcare systems to implement change and ensuring the continuous education of nursing staff to adopt best practices. The future for CNSs lies in leveraging technology to improve healthcare delivery and in leading interdisciplinary teams to tackle complex healthcare challenges.

Nurse Anesthetists (CRNAs): Leaders in Anesthesia Care

CRNAs play a pivotal role in ensuring the safety and comfort of patients undergoing procedures requiring anesthesia. The autonomy of CRNAs, particularly in rural and underserved areas, highlights the critical nature of their expertise. With advancements in anesthesia techniques and the increasing complexity of surgical procedures, CRNAs are faced with the challenge of maintaining the highest standards of care while adapting to new technologies and protocols. The expansion of their roles to include pain management represents a significant area of growth, offering opportunities to impact patient care beyond the operating room.

Nurse Midwives (CNMs): Advocates for Women's Health

CNMs embody the holistic approach to women's health care, emphasizing natural childbirth and the empowerment of women in their healthcare decisions. The challenges they face include overcoming misconceptions about midwifery care and navigating legal and regulatory barriers in different states. The future for CNMs involves expanding their practice settings beyond birthing centers to mainstream healthcare systems, where they can influence broader changes in maternity care practices. Their advocacy for women's health rights and their focus on education and preventive care position them as essential contributors to the healthcare system.

Addressing Challenges and Embracing Opportunities

Advanced practice nurses face a range of challenges, from regulatory and scope-of-practice limitations to the need for continuous education and adaptation to technological advancements. Addressing these challenges requires advocacy, research, and a commitment to lifelong learning.

Opportunities for APNs continue to grow, driven by healthcare shortages, an aging population, and an increasing emphasis on preventive care and wellness. APNs are well-positioned to lead innovations in healthcare delivery, from telehealth services to integrated care models that address the physical, mental, and social determinants of health.

The expanding roles and responsibilities of APNs are critical to the evolution of healthcare. Their advanced training, clinical expertise, and patient-centered approach enable them to address complex healthcare needs, improve patient outcomes, and lead change. As the healthcare landscape continues to evolve, APNs will play increasingly pivotal roles in shaping the future of healthcare delivery, policy, and education. This chapter not only highlights the significant impact of advanced practice nursing but also serves as a call to action for nurses to pursue advanced education and certification, underscoring the profound influence APNs can have on the healthcare landscape.

Chapter 6

The Heart and Horizon of Nursing

As we draw the curtains on this exploration of nursing, it's clear that the profession stands not merely as a career but as a calling that beckons with the promise of making a tangible difference in the lives of individuals and communities. Nursing, with its rich tapestry woven from threads of care, compassion, and clinical excellence, extends an invitation to embark on a journey of endless learning, growth, and fulfillment.

Throughout this book, we've navigated the vast landscape of nursing, from the adrenaline-fueled corridors of emergency departments to the quiet, impactful spaces of hospice care. We've ventured beyond the hospital walls into the realms of public health, research, education, and administration, uncovering the diversity and depth that nursing offers. Each chapter has served as a testament to the adaptability, resilience, and critical importance of nurses in the healthcare ecosystem.

The evolution of nursing mirrors the evolution of healthcare itself—dynamic, patient-centered, and increasingly complex. As nurses, the opportunity to specialize, advance, and lead in various settings allows us to tailor our career paths to our passions and interests. The pursuit of specialized certifications and advanced practice roles not only enhances our skill set but also elevates the standard of care we provide to our patients.

Yet, the essence of nursing transcends the technical competencies and advanced certifications. It lies in the human touch—the ability to offer solace in moments of vulnerability, to advocate tirelessly for our patients, and to lead with empathy and integrity. This essence is the beacon that guides our practice, illuminating the path toward holistic, compassionate care.

As we look to the future, the role of nurses will undoubtedly expand and evolve in response to global health challenges, technological advancements, and the shifting landscape of healthcare delivery. The demand for skilled, compassionate nursing professionals is unwavering, and the opportunities for impact are limitless.

To those who are called to this noble profession: embrace the journey with open hearts and curious minds. The path of nursing is one of lifelong learning, where each experience enriches your practice and every challenge strengthens your resolve. Remember, in the tapestry of healthcare, nurses are the vital threads that hold the fabric together, weaving the story of human resilience, care, and healing.

In closing, this book is but a gateway into the vast world of nursing—a world where passion meets purpose, where challenges transform into opportunities, and where every day offers the chance to make a difference. Let us step forward with courage, compassion, and commitment, ready to shape the future of healthcare, one patient, one community, and one innovation at a time. For in the heart of nursing lies the power to heal, to inspire, and to change the world.

www.ingramcontent.com/pod-product-compliance
Lightning Source LLC
Chambersburg PA
CBHW071021290526
45795CB00005B/1884